What to buy for baby

Sarah Hudson

Dedication

To the three people who most helped me survive the sleep deprivation that comes with a baby - Neal, my Mum and Nic. And of course to Samuel, the source of my sleep deprivation and of so many smiles.

Contents

Acknowledgments

Thanks to all my friends who found time to make suggestions for this book but especially to Nicola Bullivent, who somehow managed to find time to read everything (several times!) and make helpful suggestions while also caring for her beautiful daughter Freya.

1 Introduction

Do you think of yourself as a 'prepared' type of person? I like to – I mean, I own a torch in case of power cuts, I have a pound coin which I keep exclusively for use in supermarket trolleys and swimming pool lockers and I always carry a spare pair of tights wrapped in plastic with me to weddings as insurance against my uncanny ability to unite tights with adverse surfaces. But for some reason this day-to-day Boy Scout-esque ethos of 'Be Prepared' didn't seem to transfer very well to getting ready for baby and I really struggled to work out what I needed to buy. I'd read plenty of pregnancy/baby books, but while they were great for learning about breast-feeding, sleep-training and lochia they didn't seem to cover what you actually needed to buy for baby all that well.

This meant that when I went shopping to buy things for baby I found it hard to work out which items were 'essentials' and which were just cunningly designed to extort money out of hormonally-ravaged mums-to-be such as myself. In fact, I ended up being so indecisive about the whole thing that I put off buying anything for absolutely ages until a good friend suggested that unless I planned on fashioning baby's first outfit out of a hospital pillowcase I'd better get on and do some serious shopping.

It just so happened that this wake-up call coincided with an NCT (National Childbirth Trust) "Nearly New" sale, so with newly discovered urgency I dragged my husband along to it. The first purchase I made was a baby bath and having broken my 'buying for baby' duck I then waddled between the sale tables like a woman possessed, buying baby clothes in bulk. Emboldened by this experience we went straight from the sale to a local hypermarket where I filled a trolley with cellular blankets, sheets, muslins, mega-bags of cotton wool, baby wipes and a variety of different nappies (plus of course some chocolate, which at this point I was eating in industrial quantities).

Once we got home I did load after load of washing and then stared in wonderment at the tiny clothes drying on the airers. I felt that I was clearly on a roll so sat down and consulted Mr Google on what else I needed to buy. And this was where it all got rather confusing. What one website confidently declared was 'essential' the next dismissed as 'a waste of money', and when I turned to baby/mums forums looking for clarity things instead became even more hazy. While some things were very clear-cut (for example, I needed to buy a car seat and a cot or crib or moses basket for baby to sleep in) other things were clearly very controversial.

In the end, I didn't buy much more before baby arrived, which worked out fine(ish) except for a few minor points, such as that when he did arrive he vomited/poo-ed/wee-ed on all of his sleepsuits within the first 48 hours and it became apparent that I really needed something I could put him safely in other than his crib when I had to do things. Retrospectively, I think that overall I could have made the first few weeks a lot easier on myself, my husband (and probably my baby too) had I been smarter in what I'd bought in advance. And I would have probably wasted less money on things that actually turned out to be about as useful as a bikini in Antarctica.

So this is why I felt motivated to write this book – to share with you things I learnt belatedly that I wish someone had told me before I'd had Sam.

Now, if you've already read any books/websites about babies I'm sure you're aware that around any topic related to children there is always controversy, and any suggestions on what you should buy for baby is no different. So unfortunately this book cannot possibly be definitive; what it can be is a (hopefully very useful) guide. It is a mixture of what I've learnt, combined with what other mummies I know have taught me, blended with the opinions of literally hundreds of mums I've never met but who contributed to over

500 posts on a selection of internet forums discussing under various titles what you should and shouldn't buy for your baby.

Now it goes without saying that these mummies often disagreed – virtually every item appeared on both 'worst' and 'best' buy lists – so what this book aims to do is give you as balanced a viewpoint as possible so you can make up your own mind as to whether different items are likely to be useful to you. The inconvenient fact is that as much as it would be nice for me to simply write an authoritative list of what you need to buy, a 'one size fits all' list of things to buy for baby wouldn't actually be that useful because everyone has different homes, lifestyles and parenting wishes, all of which will impact on what should be on your personal list. And because of the huge range of options available for many items, and the uniqueness of each mum's needs, I've often ended up providing 'points to ponder' to try and guide you to the right choice for you rather than favouring one option over another.

Basically, this book is the book I wish I could've had to read before I had Sam. My hope is that when you've read it you will feel confident with what you need/want to buy so that when baby arrives you will feel you've chosen wisely and not wasted money on unnecessary items.

2 Using
"What to buy for baby"

I've divided the book into chapters with each covering a particular aspect of things you'll need to buy for baby, so you can easily dip in and out at leisure. Each chapter starts with a list of items you may wish to consider buying related to that topic, then goes on to discuss each item in more detail to help you decide if you do really want/need to buy it. In case you have "pregnancy brain" as badly as I did there is also a "Rating" under the heading for each item before the blurb about it commences. The ratings used are:

Essential – you really need this.

Advisable – you could live without this, but your life is likely to be a lot easier with it.

Optional – your decision on whether or not you want this will depend on your personal preference for the item based on your circumstances.

For some items I've also included statistics from my internet reading of 'best and worsts' on various mummy forums to try and give you an idea of how many mummies thought the item was useful versus how many thought it useless. The two main reasons I haven't included statistics for some items are:

1) Some items that are 'essential' weren't really commented on enough for me to produce statistics, probably because mums considered them too mundane or obvious to warrant typing about. Examples of items that would fall into this category include cots, nappies and vest tops.

2) Raw statistics for some items would suggest they are a 'worst' buy and not worth buying when in fact the mums writing about them on the forums really meant that the item was an inappropriate buy for them. An example of this would be the number of mums who listed 'breast pump' as a worse buy because they decided not to breast feed.

I've also tried to provide a guide of what the cheapest/most expensive price for buying the various items new is likely to be. These were all correct in Spring 2012 and came from comparing prices at five common UK high street stores (in case you're interested, they were, in alphabetical order, Asda, Boots, Mamas and Papas, Mothercare and Tesco.)

If you're thinking of buying second-hand (more about that in Chapter 12) as a guide in most cases the price should be around a third the new price.

And just in case you are already breaking into a cold sweat over how much this is all going to cost, let me sneak a few figures in here...

As of Spring 2012, if you purchased everything this book recommends as 'essential' or 'advisable' new but as cheaply as possible, you would spend around £615. If you bought as many of those items second hand as possible (because some things, such as maternity pads, really need to be new!) you'd spend around £270. And if you chose to buy only the 'essential' things, these numbers decrease to £280 and £145 respectively. So hopefully you can now begin this book feeling slightly less apprehensive about your bank balance!

3 Clothes

Sleepsuits – newborn size x 10

Sleepsuits – 0-3 months x 10

Vests – newborn size x 5

Vests – 0-3 months x 10

Cardigans x 2

Outdoor suit x 1

Hats x 3

Posh outfit x 1

Socks x 5 pairs

Sockons x 2 pairs

Mits

Napisan

Before we charge off into specifics of the items of clothing listed at the start of this chapter, just a few general points to digest that are relevant to all of them:

1) Small babies are capable of producing volumes of poo, wee and vomit that are utterly disproportionate to their size. They also seem to be able to get these various bodily fluids onto their clothes with alarming frequency. This means you are likely to be changing your newborn a lot. Actually, let me make that a LOT in capital letters. And your wiggly, and often impatient, newborn is likely to be even less thrilled about this than you. So, in order to minimize the trauma of these changes, for both baby and you, try and buy clothes that are easy to get on and off.

2) The natural progression from point 1 is that the clothes you buy for baby are going to need washing a lot, so, obvious though it seems, try and get clothes that are machine-washable. Amazingly, some baby clothes actually are hand-wash only, which almost guarantees they will hardly ever be worn, unless you are lucky enough to have a live-in maid or a partner whose secret hobby is doing hand-washing.

3) Pretty dresses with lace trims and bows look sweet on little girls, and mini-denim jeans and hooded tops make little boys look oh-so adorably like tiny grown-ups, but the reality is that for the

first couple of months your baby is going to spend a lot of their time sleeping, even during the daytime. Since their sleep sessions are going to be spontaneous and frequent, you aren't going to be changing their clothes for them (and, lets be honest, you're going to be changing them enough anyway!) With this in mind, would you be comfortable sleeping in your best party frock or hooded jumper with the hood bunched up under your neck? Or would you be happier in an all-in-one sleepsuit which is soft all over? And, thinking back to point 1, cute outfits are less easy to change than sleepsuits, so overall in the early days sleepsuits may well make both you and your newborn happier.

4) You cannot be sure what size your baby will be when born, or how quickly they will grow. My bump was consistently measuring "small", but when Sam arrived he was nearly 10lbs and wouldn't fit into any of the newborn clothes I'd bought. With this in mind, its best to make sure you initially have a small number of both newborn and 0 to 3 month sizes of clothes, and that you don't spend too much on newborn clothes which may well be worn for only a short period of time, or possibly not at all!

So with these general points in mind (hopefully, although baby-brain can make it hard to remember anything) let's move on to consider specific items...

Sleepsuits
Rating: essential
Price new: £2 to £19 each

As discussed in the preamble above, in the early weeks your baby is likely to really just need sleepsuits. Straightforward, right? Well, not quite. Because, believe it or not, there are some little variations between sleepsuits that you need to consider beyond just the colour and picture on the front. The main questions to ask yourself when looking at a sleepsuit to potentially buy are:

1. How does it fasten?

You want to be able to lie baby on it then rapidly do it up. This may seem obvious but it wasn't to me so while most sleepsuits I owned were the standard 'poppers on front, easy to do up' kind I also ended up buying some very beautiful sleepsuits with poppers up the back. Bad move. They are such hassle I only used them twice – once before I'd established what hassle they were, and once when Sam had had such a 'productive' day all his other sleepsuits were dirty. Additionally, lying on the poppers left little marks down his back, which made me feel disproportionately guilty (in fact, I may have cried. Darn hormones.)

And, even if the sleepsuit has poppers on the front, where on the front are they? Some sleepsuits have poppers down the centre and partly down both legs – these are my personal favourites (and also happily the commonest kind) as they are the easiest to get an uncooperative baby into and out of. Other sleepsuits may have poppers in a trendier 'diagonal' fashion across the body and down just one leg. These are not quite as easy to do up as you have to wrestle one leg into the suit rather than just poppering it in, but it's not much harder and the fact they often look a bit nicer helps to compensate for the extra effort.

The final common style is to just have poppers around the legs so you have to put the sleepsuit on over baby's head. This is slightly more fiddly than poppers down the front and a real problem if you happen to have a baby who hates having things pulled over their head.

2. Does it have 'feet'?

If it does, you do not need socks. This makes dressing both quicker and simpler, because if you think how difficult it is to keep adult socks in functioning pairs, just imagine what a pain baby ones will be, and that is before you get to the logistics of keeping the socks on...

3. Does it have integral mittens?

This is in no way an essential, but a few sleepsuits with cuffs that can fold over the hands as little built-in mittens can be useful for when your baby is going through a 'scratchy' stage and seems determined to make their face look like they've been dragged through a bramble patch overnight.

4. What material is it made of?

Most sleepsuits are cotton, but some are thicker "velour" type material, which may be a pro or con depending on the season.

In total you probably want around 10 sleepsuits in each size.

Vests

Rating: essential
Price new: £1 to £4 each

Vests are either worn alone (if it's hot in the summer) or under sleepsuits if it's cooler. The commonest form are short sleeved, and have nice wide necks which allow you to take them off over baby's bottom as well as over the head. If you're having a winter baby investing in vests with attractive designs on them is likely to be a bit of a waste as there will almost always be a sleepsuit covering them up, so you could save money by just buying the plain white ones (which are also easier to bleach if baby gets poo all over them...)

Vests can also be long-sleeved, which is invaluable in winter as at night baby's body and legs will be snug inside sleeping bag/under blanket but arms will likely be out getting cold so it's good to have an additional long-sleeved layer under the sleepsuit

In total you will probably want around 10 vests in each size, as on a bad day your baby may vomit/pee/poo through 5 – Sam's record was 6, having managed both a hat-trick of poos plus two vomits then a bonus wee!

Cardigans
Rating: essential
Price new: £5 to £24 each

If it's a bit chilly you'll want to own a couple of warm cardigans that are easy to slip on and off of baby. Even if in your own life you are a jumper kind of person (as I am) you'll quickly see the cardigan comes into its own for babies as it is just so much easier to put on/take off than a jumper. This is also where grandmas/elderly aunts/skilled friends can come into their own as woolly cardies can look lovely and stretch well when you are getting wiggly arms into them. However, if family members are expressing an interest in knitting for you try to persuade them to knit in a wool that is machine-washable, else you'll find you either rarely use it or you end up throwing it in the washing machine by accident and shrink it.

If you're buying from a shop it's worth trying to make sure at least one cardie is 'traditional' and doesn't have a hood on it as you won't want the hood up inside/when baby is in the car and if left down they tend to get bunched up behind baby's neck/upper back, which looks fairly uncomfortable.

Outdoor suit
Rating: advisable to essential
(depending on season baby is born in)
Price new: £15 to £35 each

Once the weather becomes colder a cardigan isn't enough so you'll need at least one outdoor suit, which is like a sleepsuit but made of warmer material. These come in a variety of designs, ranging from cute teddy bear-like suits to padded velour snowsuits. I must confess to being somewhat seduced by how cute these all looked and ended up with a one in a teddy bear design (which I loved so much I ended up owning in 3 different sizes), a cow print one, a grey bear one and a couple of thick snowsuits... I'm sure you won't be surprised to learn that some of these were barely worn, but since I bought nearly all of them cheaply second-hand I didn't feel too guilty about it!

When choosing your baby's outdoor suit think about:

• ***how cold it's likely to be*** when baby will be wearing it - mid-winter = thick, padded one, autumn = thinner one.

• ***how easy it will be to clean*** - lots of long white fur = attractive but impractical, brown padded one = less attractive (obviously depending on your personal opinion) but infinitely more practical for keeping clean.

• ***whether it has an integral hood*** or not - if it does, you won't necessarily need to find a hat when you're in a hurry to go out in milder weather.

• ***if it has built in mits*** – if it does, you won't have to worry about losing gloves.

• ***if the feet are attached or not*** – some have integral feet, whilst others have separate 'booties' for the feet... which are obviously more likely to fall off or have a little gap between them and the suit to make baby cold.

An outdoor suit with integral 'feet' is especially useful if you think you'll be using a carrier/sling lots, as carriers tend to hoick trousers not held down by feet bits up to short proportions, leaving lots of exposed, cold-looking leg.

Hats
Rating: essential
Price new: £1 to £10 each

Young babies are unable to regulate their body temperature, so since most heat is lost through the head if it's cold outside a hat is an essential. Equally, if it's summer a sunhat to protect baby's head from burning is equally important. Make sure you buy a couple and ensure they are also machine washable – if your baby gets cradle cap (and many babies do) this can be rather malodorous so you'll want to wash the hat frequently!

Posh outfit(s)
Rating: optional
Price new: £6 to £45

As explained in the introduction to this section you're unlikely to want to put baby into a 'posh' outfit very often initially but it is nice to have one (or two!) to show your baby off in on special occasions. However, since these outfits are so adorable friends/relatives may well buy them for you as gifts, so you may decide not to bother buying any for yourself and instead use your money for other more practical (but less cute) items that others won't buy for you.

Some mummies love dressing their babies up from the very beginning, but even if you think you're going to fall into this category I'd still advise not buying too many outfits to start with, partly in case you decide once baby comes along that actually the outfits are too much hassle and partly because outfits tend to be more expensive than sleepsuits so it's even more annoying if you then end up having a 'newborn' that goes straight into 0-3 month sizes, meaning they never get to wear their cute newborn outfits at all!

Socks
Rating: advisable
Price new: £0.50 to £3 per pair

Socks are vital if you have sleepsuits without feet in them, or to go with posh outfits. However, as mentioned under 'sleepsuits' they are a royal pain, so you may be wondering why I've still included so many pairs on this list. Well, the fact is that although they may be rubbish as socks they make great mittens/scratch mitts – and ironically they tend to stay on better than the items of clothing designed to be put on babies' hands. Which is vital since babies' fingernails become dagger-like surprisingly quickly and they are somewhat slow to learn that raking their fingernails across their face is not a good idea, and it can be embarrassing taking your baby to baby group looking like they've just lost a fight with a bad-tempered cat.

As an aside, it's also a good idea to buy a mesh laundry bag to wash these in (if you don't already own one) as they are so small they tend to get lost inside other items of washing/magically disappear within the washing machine.

Sockons

Rating: optional
Price new: around £3 per pair

Sockons are ingenious little elasticated items which hold socks in place. If baby is going to be wearing socks on a regular basis these are invaluable to stop you having to spend your time putting socks back on, or getting halfway round the supermarket and realising that yet again baby is recreating the Cinderella story with their sock and no Prince Charming is going to bring it back.

Mits

Rating: optional
Price new: £1 to £2 per pair

Mits are useful for stopping baby scratching

themselves and also for keeping their hands warm in cooler weather. However, most mums (myself included) find they are utterly rubbish at staying on, so as mentioned above using baby socks instead is a good alternative – not only do they stay on better, but they can also be used for their intended function as socks when no longer needed as mits!

Napisan
Rating: advisable
Price new: around £2.50 a box

Napisan is something that could almost be used as a test to see if someone has had a baby: those that have know about it, those that haven't, don't. So, to promote you to the 'in the know' group, let me tell you about it...it's a 'magic' powder that you can put in with your usual powder when you wash baby clothes to help remove some of the more stubborn stains (particularly poo). It is not a miracle cure but it is very good (and safe to be used on baby clothes) and napisan, combined with drying in sunlight (another top secret mummy tip for getting rid of poo stains) salvaged many of Sam's white vests and sleepsuits in the early months.

4 Sleeping

Moses basket or crib
Sheets for crib/moses
 basket/cot x 4
Cellular blankets x 2
Sleeping bags x 3
Cot
Night lights
Dummies x 4
Mobile
Baby monitor
Swaddle cloth

Moses basket or Crib

Rating: optional
Price new: £25 (basic moses basket) to above £400 (posh crib)

Most babies start life sleeping in a moses basket or crib (after having probably initially slept in the fish-tank type cots you have in hospital maternity wards). Moses baskets/cribs are smaller than a cot so feel more like the womb, meaning many babies feel safer in them and so find it easier to sleep. The smaller size also means they are more likely to be able to fit into your bedroom than a cot. There are two main benefits of being able to have baby in your bedroom initially:

1.you have less far to go during the night to feed/soothe your baby

2.research suggests babies who sleep in their parent's room are at lower risk of cot death

Reasons you may decide not to bother to purchase a moses basket/crib include that babies tend to grow out of them quickly (in general within the first 2 to 3 months) which can make it difficult to justify spending money on one, and some babies just never like the 'smallness' of them and so may refuse to ever settle in one... for example, my baby Sam was always a fan of flailing his arms around so never slept well in his crib as he kept waking himself by hitting the side (to be honest he was never great at sleeping in his cot either, but at least when he did get to sleep in that he didn't wake himself due to his hands colliding with the sides!).

If you do decide to invest in a moses basket or crib and need to decide which to go for, the main advantages of buying a moses basket over a crib is that it is more portable, so during the day you can move baby from room to room with you while they are asleep in it, and also that a moses basket is likely to be cheaper to buy.

Another possibility if you don't want to buy either but want something your baby can sleep in during the day and you can move around the home with you is to buy a pram with a carrycot part which could be used for this purpose.

Another alternative if you wanted somewhere for baby to sleep downstairs during the day but didn't want to buy a moses basket or crib would be to buy a travel cot with a bassinet included (=bit that goes in the travel cot to make it like a crib rather than a cot) and put this up in your living room. This could be less of a waste of money (as you can use it as a travel cot/playpen once you no longer need a downstairs 'crib') but be careful to make sure you have one that will fit in the room you intend to use it in, as travel cots can be quite big. If you fancy reading more about travel cots now, have a sneaky peep forward to Chapter 8 where they are discussed in more detail.

So what do mums who have bought moses baskets think of them? Well, on the internet forums the popularity of moses baskets on the best/worst buy lists was divisive – over 10% of posters listed it as a worst buy (commonly lamenting how quickly their baby outgrew it) while 5% of posters mentioned it on their best buy lists (often stating how handy it was to be able to carry their sleeping baby around the house with them). So once again, it's up to you to decide which group you think you'll agree with!

Sheets for crib/moses basket/cot
Rating: essential
Price new: £5 to £15 each

Sheets for crib/moses basket/cot/pram are boring but important items. Make sure you buy a few (probably 4) as they are likely to get coated in vomit/urine/poo on a fairly frequent basis. Just like with adult beds you can buy fitted sheets, which are obviously easier to change than traditional flat ones.

Cellular blankets
Rating: essential
Price new: £5 to £18

Cellular blankets are blankets that are slightly 'mesh-like' in design, meaning that even if baby managed to pull one over themselves they should still be able to breathe. It's advisable to buy at least a couple of these as they can serve multiple purposes, such as:

- over baby at night when newborn to keep warm (and beyond if you decide not to use sleeping bags)
- over baby in the pram/pushchair if it's chilly
- over baby in bouncy chair if there's a draught
- as a swaddle in colder weather
- as a small mat to lie baby on at baby groups

However, many mums on the internet forums regretted the number of cellular blankets they bought. One of the common reasons given for this was that once their babies were in sleeping bags at night they no longer needed cellular blankets for nighttime and they preferred other types of blankets for daytime uses. It might therefore be an idea not to buy too many... I had 4 and I'm fairly certain I never even used at least one of them, and they haven't come out of their drawer at all since Sam was around 2 months old.

Sleeping bags

Rating: most mums would say 'essential', but you could class them as merely 'advisable' as you can use cellular blankets instead.
Price new: £12 to £65

I had never heard of baby sleeping bags before I had Sam, but quite frankly I now have no idea how I (or he!) would have coped without them – and I'm definitely not alone, as they were the second most commonly mentioned item on the internet 'best buy' lists with 92 mums loving them enough to recommend them and only 3 mums posting that they regretted purchasing them.

With such positive feedback you'll not be surprised to learn that there are multiple benefits to using baby sleeping bags over blankets:

1. Baby can't kick the sleeping bag off during the night and then get cold (and so cry and wake you up)

2. Baby can stay in the sleeping bag while you are feeding her during the night so when you put her back down she isn't going onto a cold sheet, meaning she is likely to settle more quickly

3. Baby can't slip down inside a sleeping bag while they can slip under a blanket, meaning a sleeping bag should be safer

4. Baby's feet are safely contained within the

sleeping bag so less likely to get stuck through the sides of the cot (although I have a fabulous photo of Sam still managing to get both feet through the sides of his cot despite being in a sleeping bag!)

5. Baby's hands are outside the sleeping bag while torso and legs are inside so they are less able to scratch themselves (this is particularly relevant if your baby has eczema)

However, it must be noted that sleeping bags have a minimum weight requirement to ensure baby can't slip down inside, so depending on how big your newborn is you may not be able to use them until they are a bit older.

When you are choosing a sleeping bag, just like when choosing sleepsuits, look at how it fastens. Most have zips, which are fast, easy and exactly what you want to be doing up in the semi-darkness at 3am (if you have to be doing anything up at all, as obviously it is far more preferable to be sleeping at 3am). Other sleeping bags fasten with a line of poppers, which is more fiddly and time-consuming and therefore definitely less preferable.

An additional small detail when choosing a sleeping bag is if it fastens with a zip, does the zip fasten from the bottom up to the top, or from the top down to the bottom? The relevance of this becomes apparent if you need to change baby during the night. If you prefer to get baby out of the sleeping bag to change her its best if the zip fastens from bottom to top, as you don't have to completely separate the 2 parts of the zip to take the sleeping bag off, whereas if it fastens from the top to the bottom you have to completely separate the zip to take the sleeping bag off, and then coordinate re-joining the two halves when you put it back on.

These may seem like pernickety details, but when you are trying to do up the sleeping bag in the early hours while sleep-deprived you will curse yourself if it's not as easy as possible, especially if you end up taking so long that your previously just dopey baby wakes up 'properly' and then decides its play time...

The other thing to remember is that just like adult duvets sleeping bags come in different 'togs' (the commonest being 1 for summer and 2.5 for winter) so make sure you buy the right tog for the season baby is born in.

Cot

Rating: essential
Price new: cot: £60 to over £800;
mattress £18 to over £300

A cot is obviously essential (unless you are planning on entirely co-sleeping, in which case feel free to skip this bit.) Many versions are available, from basic "just a cot" to types which have built-in storage underneath and can be transformed into a toddler bed at a later date. The main things to consider when choosing a cot are:

• *Is the base height of the cot adjustable?* If so, you can have baby at a higher level when they are little so you don't have to bend down so far to pick baby up but then are able to lower it once baby is bigger so they can't climb out (quick hint for the future: make sure you lower the base in time. Sam progressed to pulling himself up with surprising speed and we had literally only dropped the base the night before he achieved this milestone...)

• *Does the cot has 'drop sides'?* This might be helpful if you aren't very tall and worry you might find it difficult to pick baby up from the bottom of the cot or if you are prone to back problems

• *Can the cot be converted into a 'toddler bed' at a later date?* The benefits of buying a cot that have this conversion option are firstly saving money (as you won't need to buy a toddler bed too) and secondly it may make the transition from cot to toddler bed less daunting for the child, and therefore less traumatic for both them and you!

All cots sold new in the UK will conform to strict standards regarding the materials used, the width between the bars and the depth from the base to the top. If you buy a second-hand one check when and where it was originally bought to check that it would have also conformed to these standards when new.

Most cots are sold separate to the mattress, and obvious though it sounds make sure you get the right size mattress for the cot you have (I put this in as when I went to buy a mattress I just thought I'd be able to purchase one in 'cot size' without thinking that cots are not all one size... yet another 'fail' I'll blame on my pregnancy brain). It's also a good idea to either buy a mattress with a removable, washable cover, or to buy one of these separately to protect it from the delightful bodily fluids your baby will try and saturate it with.

Even if you get given a cot second hand (as I did, thank you Sarah G) you should really get a new mattress, as official advice recommends a new mattress for each baby to decrease the risk of cot death.

Night lights
Rating: optional
Price new: around £8 per pack of 2

After purchasing my plug-in night light (in fact two!) the number of stubbed toes I suffered whilst attending to Sam at night decreased substantially... I really wish I'd bought them sooner! Other benefits to having night lights include allowing the parent who is awake to see what they are doing without having to turn on a bright light that disturbs the parent who is trying to sleep, and in a similar vein allows you to feed a partially-awake baby without completely waking them up and making them think "ooo, bright light, it's daytime!" (and so hopefully meaning they will quickly go back to sleep again, rather than decide it's playtime.)

Personally I found that a dull night light that stayed on continuously in the room Sam was sleeping in was very useful, as it meant I could see enough to feed him but it was still dark enough for him to sleep, and then when he moved to his own room I also had a brighter one in the hallway to help me navigate from our room to his without incident/injury. It might be worth you seeing how bright baby's room/your hallway are at night before you baby arrives, so you can assess how many/what brightness of nightlights would work best for you.

Dummies

Rating: optional
Price new: from £1 each

Dummies provoke such great debate that I feel I should be writing this section whilst wearing a flak jacket and waving a white flag. You'll find some parents are venomously opposed to them, whilst others are equally passionately in love with them. Obviously its up to you to make up your own mind which camp you wish to belong to (and switching camps is definitely allowed!), but it's worth knowing that many mums find that a dummy can be invaluable in helping to soothe a tired baby to sleep. I personally started using one with Sam for naps/sleeping when I realised that he was using me (or more specifically my breast) as a living dummy. Which was lovely when he was little (and probably good for increasing my milk production) but less great as he got a bit older and I needed to be able to get on and do dull things like housework when he was asleep.

Additionally, current research suggests a baby sleeping with a dummy is at less risk of cot death, which is clearly an advantage and also a great fact to be able to quote to people who may disapprove of your decision to use one.

If you do decide to use dummies, firstly note that they come in different sizes for different ages (yet another of those things that I just didn't realise...) and secondly note that you need to choose whether you go for an 'orthodontic' or 'cherry' style one. The difference is that orthodontic ones are flatter, and are, as their name suggests, supposed to be better for teeth, while 'cherry' ones are the more traditional round ones. Whichever one you choose, you may find your baby has other ideas and will only accept the other type, or may decide they don't want one at all! Also, babies love 'shaking things up', so after a month of a dummy being the magic solution to Sam not sleeping he utterly refused one for over a month, and then it was suddenly like a magic solution again... and then he made his final decision that he didn't want a dummy anymore (and shortly afterwards recruited his thumb to fill the role left vacant by the dummy)... so don't be surprised if your baby's feelings about their dummy are as divided as your own may be!

It is also worth remembering that if you are breast-feeding you should avoid using a dummy until baby has definitely got the hang of latching and feeding, to avoid 'nipple confusion'.

Mobiles
Rating: optional
Price new: £10 to £50

A newborn is unlikely to be interested in a mobile (it is too far away for their limited vision and doesn't fit into their life plan of feed, poo, scream, sleep) but once baby is a few weeks old a mobile may be used to:
- calm a distressed baby
- temporarily amuse/distract baby while whilst

you do something (such as managing to pee!)

• help as part of a sleep time routine

Mums seem to be very divided on mobiles – similar numbers list them on their 'best buy' list as those that put them on their 'worst buy' list. This may be due to the differing attitudes of different babies to them (for example some babies are stimulated rather than relaxed by them, which is hopeless if you purchased the mobile hoping for it to help with the bedtime routine), or possibly due to the type of mobiles being used – for example, 'traditional' wind-up mobiles which often only play for around 2 minutes are unlikely to allow you much time to do something, while 'battery' ones often play for 20 minutes – which if your baby is amused by it for that long is likely to be very useful in terms of getting things done!

From my personal mobile experience I'd put mobiles on both the best and worst buy lists. My mobile use started with a wind-up mobile which played for 1 minute and 55 seconds and which amused 2 month old Sam fantastically, so I used to get my washing up done in 100 second bursts before running to wind the mobile again. This would have temporarily placed mobiles on my best buy list, because although not ideal at least it meant I could (sort of) do my washing up. However, even in my sleep-deprived not-thinking-straight state this 100 second burst approach seemed a suboptimal arrangement so I then bought a (ridiculously expensive) battery mobile that boasted a 20 minute playtime, multiple songs and noises, remote control and snazzy lightshow as well as the 'normal' mobile part. Sam hated it, was never entertained by any of the songs and it was a complete waste of money and at the time would have zoomed straight to the top of my worst-buy list.

So, after that slightly disheartening anecdote which illustrates how unpredictable babies' responses to mobiles can be, what things might you want to consider when choosing a mobile if you do decide to go for it? Below are a few points to help guide you:

• *How long does the music play for?* As mentioned above, a couple of minutes is unlikely to be that helpful for anything

• *What is the music?* The second mobile I bought had tunes that I discovered I absolutely detested, which might have been just about bearable had Sam been amused by it but it turned out he felt the same way about the tunes as I did!

• *Does it have options other than music*, such as 'heartbeat' for young babies or 'white noise' to help with sleep?

• *Is there a volume control option?*

• *How is it powered* – batteries or wind up?

• *Does it come with a remote control?* This

may seem incredibly lazy, but a mobile with a remote control may be able to reduce the number of times you get out of bed (if your baby will resettle with the mobile alone) and also means you can turn it on without baby seeing you, which may also increase the chances of baby resettling

• ***Does it have a lightshow?*** If it does, it might be useful right into toddler years.

And once you've chosen one, I'd recommend crossing your fingers that it has the effect you desire on your baby!

Baby monitor
Rating: advisable
Price new: from £20 to over £150

Baby monitors are fairly vital if you live in a larger house and might not be able to hear baby in their cot while you are in another room, and even if you live in a small flat you may want a monitor for the reassurance it offers. They come in a huge range of shapes, sizes and prices, with an utterly dazzling array of possible features – some have built-in light shows, lullabies, timers, night-lights, thermometers, talk-back options... The important thing to remember when choosing one is that you are buying it to be a baby monitor, so don't be seduced by other features on it that you don't really need (and could probably buy cheaply as a separate product if you really wanted them).

Fundamentally monitors now come with 3 'surveillance' types:

• **Basic audio monitors** – these are the traditional type of monitor with which you can hear baby only. If you opt for one of these make sure it is digital as the clarity of sound is so much better than the cheaper (and now uncommon) 'classic' monitors

• **Audio plus video monitors** – allow you to see as well as hear your baby, which potentially has the benefit of allowing you to see why baby is crying before you go to them

• **Movement monitors** – these are mats that go under the mattress and alert you if baby hasn't moved/breathed for a set period of time. They are usually sold in conjunction with either an audio or video monitor. The idea is that they alert you if baby has stopped breathing (which an audio or video monitor wouldn't) so you could act fast. However, there is currently no evidence they decrease the risk of cot death, so it is debatable whether they are worthwhile, although some mums swear they would not be without the reassurance these provide.

Once you've decided on the 'type' of monitor you

want to buy, other things to consider include:

• *How long the battery time is* on the 'parent unit' (= the bit you listen to) ?

• *How small/light is the parent unit?* This is important since you may want to carry it around with you

• *What is the range of the monitor?* This is more relevant if you live in a big house or plan on taking the parent unit out into the garden

• *How long is the warranty?* This is especially important if you are buying an expensive model

• *Does it has a 'talkback' option,* in which you can talk to the baby from the parent unit? This can be useful if you are lucky enough to have a baby who can be soothed just by hearing your voice, and can also be used to turn the baby monitor into a 'walkie-talkie' if you are with baby and your other half has the parent unit

• *Does it have a 'finder' option* in case you forget where you have put down the parent unit? (surprisingly easy to do with 'baby brain'!)

• *Is it easy to tell if it's on and at what volume it is on at*? Sounds obvious but my baby monitor doesn't show what volume it is on at so on occasion I've managed to decrease the volume to 'mute' accidentally and not realised until Sam was crying loudly enough for me to hear without the monitor...

• **_Does the monitor have any 'added extras'_** that you actually really want (such as temperature display, timer, night light, lullabies...) but as mentioned above, remember that you may be able to buy these options separately more cheaply.

Swaddle cloth
Rating: optional
Price new: £10 to £25

Some babies don't like the 'bigness' of the world after the cocoon-like environment of the womb and so like to be swaddled to recreate the secure, snug environment they enjoyed for 9 months. Also, newborns are not yet aware that their flailing upper limbs belong to them, so can be quite scared by these random 'things' that flash past their face/into their face periodically, and by swaddling you can keep them under control.

Swaddling a baby can therefore help calm a baby, help them sleep, and can also be useful to when feeding as it keeps all their limbs in check!

Now any sheet/blanket can in theory be used to swaddle a baby, and the midwives in the hospital make the swaddling process look effortless, but managing it at home, when sleep-deprived, hormonally challenged and distracted by baby screams can be harder. Investing in a specially-designed swaddle cloth or blanket can therefore make a midwife-standard swaddle easier to achieve. When looking at options look to see how it works (some fold by clever design of bits of material, while other 'pods' have a zip) and check the material it's made from isn't too heavy, as one potential danger of swaddling is overheating your baby.

5 Changing baby

Changing mat
Changing table
Nappies x 70
Cotton wool
Wipes x 6 packs
Nappy bags
Nappy bin
Zinc oxide cream
Changing bag

Changing mat
Rating: advisable
Price new: £7 to £30

A baby changing mat is not an essential – you could use a towel instead – but since a changing mat is relatively inexpensive to buy and you are likely to be using it at least ten times a day for the first few months it is probably a very sound investment. The main advantage of a 'proper' changing mat over just using a towel or similar is that a changing mat should be padded, which makes it more comfortable for baby and also means you're less likely to accidentally bang baby's head when putting them down in a hurry to change a poo-ey nappy!

When choosing a changing mat, apart from checking how padded it is, also check what the cover is made of. Most changing mats are covered in plastic, which is perfect as it makes them easy to wipe clean after any accidents. If you do decide to buy one which has a fabric cover, make sure it is removable and machine-washable (especially if you have a little boy, as they seem to be particularly talented at weeing as soon as their nappy is removed!).

Some changing mats are molded to have raised sides on the two long edges to decrease the risk of baby rolling off which some mums find useful, but since baby should never be left on a changing table alone anyway the overall benefit of raised edges is a little debatable. The final major difference between the various changing mats on the market tends to just be the design on them, which is simply a matter of personal preference.

Changing table
Rating: optional
Price new: cot-top changers from £30; changing stations from to £80; upper end of ranges over £300

Having just discussed how even a changing mat isn't essential, a changing table is absolutely not essential – in fact, many parents prefer to change their babies on the floor as there is nowhere for baby to fall to if they wiggle off the mat! However, my epic internet-forum post investigation suggests that for every mum who put 'changing table' on their worst-buy list, three mums put it on their 'best buy' list. Common reasons given for a changing table being a 'best buy' were that it saved their back, or it helped them protect their c-section scar, or it was useful to have everything in the same place. So basically a changing table should put baby at a more comfortable height to be changed and help ensure everything you need is to hand.

Versions of changing tables include:

- *A dedicated 'changing unit'* that is designed specifically for the job of changing baby, with space for the changing mat on top then storage space underneath designed with nappies/wipes in mind. The disadvantage of this type of changing table is once your baby outgrows needing it it is not necessarily very easily adapted to another use.

- *A chest of drawers with a part sitting on top that is a bit like an oversized tray* that makes it big enough to put a changing mat on. This part can then be removed once you no longer need a changing table, leaving you with a normal chest of drawers to use.

- *A 'changing tray' that fits across the top of the cot,* sitting on the bars on either side. The advantages of this type are that they don't take up additional space in the room and are relatively cheap.

However, it is worth bearing in mind that although a changing table might be extremely useful initially, once your baby becomes proficient at rolling and starts to view nappy changing time as an opportunity to develop their muscles by fighting you it is far safer to change them on the floor instead. This means that whatever you buy will likely only be used for 6 to 8 months maximum.

Nappies
Rating: essential
Price new: disposables from around 8p each; reusable starter packs from around £50

Your first choice as you enter the wonderful world of nappies is whether you want to use washable (= reusable) nappies or disposable nappies. This choice could be a huge topic on its own, but just briefly the main benefits of washable nappies are:

• overall they are cheaper than disposables (after a fairly hefty initial outlay)

• they are generally felt to be better for the environment

while the main benefits of disposable nappies are:

• there is no need to wash them = less work

• if you are out you can just bin the dirty nappy rather than having to carry it home to wash it

In theory there is now very little to separate the two types in terms of ease of use (excluding the need to wash afterwards), effectiveness as a nappy or likelihood of nappy rash.

If you are considering washable nappies I'd advise reading up as much on the internet as possible/finding support groups/seeing where you can get trial packs, as initial outlay for these can run into hundreds of pounds so you want your decision to be the right one, and the information you need to make this is beyond the scope of this book.

If you decide to go for disposables, remember that a newborn will get through around 10 nappies a day so you'll need to stock up more than you might imagine (at least 70 as a minimum) before baby arrives. There are many different brands to choose from, and unfortunately it isn't as simple as 'X brand is the best' as different brands suit different babies. I would therefore advise initially getting a pack each of several different brands to see which one seems best for your baby.

Cotton wool
Rating: optional
Price: around £1 per 100 balls

Cotton wool can be used with plain water as a gentle way to clean baby's bottom. The alternative is to use baby wipes. The advantages of cotton wool are that it is cheaper and debatably better for baby's bottom. The main disadvantage is that it is slightly less convenient than using wipes, especially when out.

Initially I'd suggest not buying too much of it just in case like me your good intentions of using

which can be invaluable in keeping your home smelling fresh rather than of 'eau de dirty baby nappy.'

Nappy bin
Rating: optional
Price: from around £7.50 (often on special offer) to around £35; cartridge refills around £5 (should last around a month)

If you live in a city where rubbish is only collected fortnightly, you may well have amassed a pile of around 140 nappies by the time the binmen visit. If you have an outside bin this may not be a problem, but if you live in a small flat with no outside bin this could be quite a (smelly) issue. In the world of internet mummy forums nappy bins seem to be another one of those divisive buys – for every mummy who put them on their 'best buy' list, 2 listed them as a 'worst buy.' Now this could be because of the different home situations (for example, the mum in the top floor flat might be listing them as a best buy while the mum with easy access to an outside bin might think it a worst buy) or because of differing effectiveness of different models.

So, while many mums (myself included) manage

just fine with a normal bin and fragranced nappy bags, others couldn't live without their special nappy bin – and as one of my good mummy friends put it "the nappy bin just makes it that little bit easier. And if I'm going to get my other half to do any nappies, it needs to be as easy as possible..."

If you do decide to get a specialized nappy bin, remember that many require 'cartridges' to work and these can be ruinously expensive, so look into this before buying – it can be a bit like buying a cheap printer for your computer and then discovering the ink cartridges cost almost as much as the printer did. Another thing to be aware of is that both nappy bins and cartridges are often on special offer so this is an item that it definitely pays to shop around for.

Zinc Oxide Cream
Rating: optional
Price: around £2.50

Zinc oxide cream (brand names include Sudocrem) is a superb cream to treat both nappy rash, which many babies will suffer from at some point, or eczema, which again will afflict many babies. It may therefore be a good idea to have a pot of this stashed away ready for when it might be needed.

As an added benefit, it can also be used on mum's sore hands (from repeated washing after changing baby) and some people swear by its ability to treat spots, which may be useful as post-pregnancy hormones temporarily make your skin behave like it is a teenager again.

Changing bag
Rating: advisable
Price: from £15 to over £200

When you go out with baby you will need to take (as a minimum) nappies, a changing mat, wipes/cotton wool and something to put the dirty nappies in. And if you have a baby like mine, probably a change of baby clothes too. It's up to you whether you want to pop all these items in a carrier bag and slot them into whichever 'normal' bag you are taking out with you, or whether you fancy treating yourself to a dedicated changing bag.

If you decide to buy a changing bag, things to consider when choosing one include:

- *Is it waterproof?*
- *Can it be washed/ wiped clean?*
- *How is it carried* – backpack, shoulder bag – and does it have straps to attach to pram?
- *Does it have separate areas for dirty and clean items?*

- ***Is there somewhere safe to keep purse, keys and phone?***
- ***Is it a design dad will carry too?!***
- ***Does it come with a changing mat?*** If so, is it a good size/is it padded?
- If you're spending lots on the bag– ***could it be used as a normal bag afterwards?***

Another possibility which sits between the 'just stuff it all in a carrier bag' option and the 'splurge on a specialized bag' choice is to buy a 'changing pouch' that you can put into any of your existing bags. Changing pouches fold out into a changing mat and have a small inbuilt pocket to hold a couple of nappies, some wipes and nappy bags. The advantages are that they are small, so can go into existing bags/bottoms of prams, they are easily transferrable from one bag to another and they are relatively cheap (costing from around £10). The main disadvantage is that you can't fit many nappies in them, so if your baby is having a 'productive' day you might find yourself running out of supplies.

6 Feeding Baby

Bottles and teats x 4

Steriliser

Bottle cleaning brush

Formula

Breast pump

Nipple cream

Bibs x 5

Feeding pillow

Bottle warmer

Bottles and teats
Rating: advisable to essential (depending on if you are breast or formula feeding)
Price new: between £3 and £10 each

Before I had Sam I would have thought Dr Brown was a local GP, Nam maybe a type of fruit and Tommee Tipee a cartoon character. Now however I know they are all brands of bottles, and there are many more brands too... Medela, Avent, Nuk... In fact, the range of bottles and teats available on the market is utterly bewildering and the first time I went to buy one from the local chemist I stood in front of the row of shelves containing the incredible selection of bottles and felt completely confused as to which I should buy. And unfortunately, just like nappies, there is no simple answer as to which brand is best so I while I can't give you a definitive answer, hopefully the following paragraphs can give you some guidance so when you confront the selection you feel slightly less confused than I did!

Just like we all have different favourite mugs or glasses, different babies like different bottles... but unfortunately while we may tolerate drinking our lemonade from a wine glass, or our wine from a tumbler, if your baby doesn't like a particular bottle (or more likely the teat that comes with that bottle) they may refuse to drink from it at all. So how can you know what bottle your baby will like? Unfortunately you can't, and as with many things in life "sod's law" applies and so will guarantee that if you buy lots of one brand of bottle before baby arrives, baby will decide they definitely do NOT like that brand, so it may be better to just buy a couple to start with to see how you get on with them.

A few pointers to help you choose your first bottles and teats are:

• In general if you are planning to switch between breast and bottle feeding a 'broader' teat will be better for your baby as it will more closely resemble the way they are used to feeding than the classic 'narrow' teats. Brands with broader teats include Tommee Tipee.

• Teats all come in different flow rates to match how fast different sized babies are likely to want to drink, so when initially buying make sure you read the box to get the right flow rate for a newborn.

• With most brands the bottle part comes in different sizes, for example Tommee Tippee ones come in 150ml/5oz, 260ml/9oz and 340ml/11oz, while Dr Browns come in 60ml/2oz, 120ml/4oz and 240ml/8oz. If this is the case with the brand you choose, it may be a good idea to go for bottle parts that are hold at least 6oz as it is likely baby will need this volume each feed within a

few months and if you've bought all 4oz bottles they will no longer be big enough for a whole feed and will therefore be fairly useless.

• ***Special 'anti-colic' bottles exist*** and some mums find these really helpful if their baby seems colic-prone. They tend to be more expensive to buy, and in some cases more fiddly to wash up, so initially you may decide to avoid them but it's worth bearing them in mind in case of future need.

If you discover you have a fussy baby who doesn't like the first brand you try, see if any of your friends with babies have different brands of bottle you can borrow for a 'trial' to potentially save you spending a small fortune building up a collection of different bottles your baby has deemed 'unacceptable.' I have a whole cupboard shelf displaying the various brands Sam decided weren't right for him, and so at 6 months of age he ended up going straight from breast-feeding to sippy cups...

Steriliser

Rating: essential (in some form) if using bottles
Price new: sterilising fluid from around £2; electric steam sterilisers from around £20 to £50; microwave

sterilisers from around £10 to £30

Sterilising bottles is very important as bacteria find milk a particularly agreeable breeding ground. This is the case regardless of whether the milk is expressed breast milk or formula, although if formula is the Hilton/Ritz of bacteria breeding grounds, expressed breast milk would be the Travelodge/Premier Inn in terms of how keen bacteria are to stay there. Either way, if you're using bottles you need a method of sterilizing them. Broadly speaking, your options are:

1. Buy nothing new and opt for the age-old 'boiling' method of sterilization.

This involves submerging the bottles and teats in a large pan of boiling water, boiling for ten minutes then allowing to cool and *eh voila* sterilized bottles. The advantage of this method is obviously you don't have to purchase anything new. The disadvantages are:

- not all bottles can be boiled
- frequent boiling is likely to decrease the lifespan of the bottles, especially the teats
- it's time-consuming as you have to keep an eye on the boiling saucepan and then wait for the bottles to cool
- it's potentially a fire hazard if you get

distracted by baby and the pan boils dry
• it's potentially dangerous as at some point you may end up with baby and boiling water in close proximity

2. Buy a big plastic tub and some sterilizing solution/tablets and become an advocate of cold water sterilization

Cold water sterilization is fairly straightforward: you take a plastic container/bucket/clean ice-cream tub, fill it with cold water, add either sterilizing solution or tablets in a quantity determined by the amount of water you've used, then submerge everything you want to be sterilized in it and leave it for half an hour. Items will then remain sterile in the water for 24 hours, and when you want to use a bottle you simply take it out, wash off the solution with cooled boiled water and use.

Advantages to this method are:
• low initial outlay for equipment
• cheap to use once sterilizing fluid/tub bought
• keeps items sterile for 24 hours
• easy to take travelling

Disadvantages to this method are:
• slow – half an hour is a long time if you have a hungry baby waiting

• needing to wash off the fluid with cooled boiled water when you remove bottles from the tub adds an extra step/hassle compared to other methods which allow you to use the bottle straight away

• splashes of the solution may bleach your clothes

• can leave bottles smelling of chemicals

3. Buy an electric steam sterilizer

This is a blissfully simple method: add tap water to your electric steam steriliser, place your bottles in it, switch it on then come back 5 to 8 minutes later and you have bottles ready to use!

Advantages:
• very easy to use
• quick – 5 to 8 minutes depending on the model

Disadvantages:
• initially more expensive to buy
• quite bulky to take travelling with you
• bottles only stay sterile for 6 hours in most models; some new models keep bottles sterile for 24 hours

4. Buy a microwave steam steriliser

This is yet another fabulously simple method, essentially very similar to the electric stream sterilizer but, well, using a microwave instead. Add tap water to it, put in your bottles, pop in the microwave and in 3 to 5 minutes you'll have sterile, ready to use bottles.

Advantages:
• very easy to use
• quickest method of sterilization
• keeps items sterile for up to 24 hours
• some units can 'double up' as a cold-water sterilisation tub

Disadvantages:
• initially more expensive to buy
• cannot use to sterilise metal items
• need to make sure it fits in your microwave

So there you go. Which you go for will depend on your budget, how often you will need to be sterilising bottles and of course your personal preference.

Bottle cleaning brush
Rating: essential if using bottles
Price new: £3 to £6

Without a bottle cleaning brush it is very hard to get bottles and teats properly clean, and getting them properly clean is obviously important to avoid bits of old milk being left in the nooks and crannies for bacteria to breed on. The good news is that although different brands of bottles try to sell you their own branded cleaning brush any will work just as well, so if you end up using different brands of bottle you should still be fine with just one brush.

Formula
Rating: advisable
Price: ready-made from around 60p per 200ml; powdered formula from £7.99 a box.

Formula milk comes either in powdered form, which you then have to mix with cooled boiled water to make up the milk, or 'premixed' form, which is ready to use. The advantage of the premixed form is obviously convenience. The disadvantage, predictably enough, is that it's a lot more expensive.

If you are planning on formula-feeding make

sure you have some before you go into labour as many hospitals now won't provide it, so you'll need to take it with you. And even if you're planning on exclusively breast-feeding, having one box of ready-made formula tucked away can provide reassurance – I remember at the end of Sam's first week sending my husband off to buy some late on a Friday night as I was just shattered and wanted to know there was something there he could give him if needed (retrospectively my husband recalls this as the moment he really knew his world had changed: instead of standing in the wine section on a Friday evening pondering red or white, he was in the baby aisle debating whether to go with Cow and Gate or Aptamil!)

Make sure you get formula that is suitable from newborn (different types exist for older babies) and also bear in mind that each brand of formula has a slightly different taste, so if your baby doesn't seem to get on with one you can try another.

Breast pump
Rating: advisable if breast feeding
Price new: manual from around £20; electric from £50

I hadn't bought a breast-pump before Sam was born, but it ended up being an emergency buy on day 3 – he was born with a tongue-tie which made breast-feeding difficult, meaning my breasts ballooned to comedy beach-postcard proportions as the poor lad just couldn't get enough milk out. And although their size may have appeared amusing, the pain from them most certainly wasn't.

However, even had breast-feeding been going swimmingly, I would have still purchased a breast pump. This is because although I planned to exclusively breast feed I still wanted to be able to leave Sam with someone else occasionally and for them to be able to give him breast milk, and I wanted to make sure Sam would accept a bottle when I wanted to move on from breast-feeding (this was the plan; sadly Sam decided he did not agree with this and steadfastly refused to take a bottle, but hey, we tried hard and spent many hours pumping milk to keep trying different bottles...)

I'd therefore summarise the reasons that as a breast-feeding mum you might want a breast-pump as:

• to be able to express milk so someone else can feed baby, for example if you want to go out for an evening or if you want dad to be able to do the occasional feed so you can catch up with sleep

• to be able to bottle-feed a baby with expressed milk yourself to try and make sure they won't refuse a bottle when you might want them to take one when they're older

- to be able to express milk while you are apart from baby (for example if you go back to work) to keep your supply up
- to empty some milk from your breasts if they become uncomfortable (but note that this should be done sparingly as it will ultimately encourage the breasts to make more milk, and hence hurt more)
- to help increase your supply if baby isn't nursing much for any reason
- to help manage mastitis (infection of the breast) as regular pumping will help milk move.

The alternative to using a breast-pump to express milk is to hand-express. The disadvantages of this are that it takes far longer and requires more attention, whereas pumping milk with an electric pump just needs one hand holding the pump to your breast and milk will come out faster. Note the word 'electric' – unless you are particularly masochistic do not be tempted by manual breast pumps as these require impressive hand muscles to be used for any period of time.

When buying a pump, the following should be considered:

- ***Manual or electric?*** Manual is harder to use, but quieter and cheaper to buy – however, the only mums I know who bought manual ones ended up buying an electric one as well, so think carefully about whether it would really be cheaper in the long run.

• *'Single' pump or 'twin' pumps?* Twin pumps extract milk from both breasts simultaneously, while single ones (as the name suggests) just do one at a time. Twin pumps are quicker, but may make you feel (and look!) even more like a human cow than a single pump, while single pumps are more usual and considerably cheaper but take longer to collect milk.

• *How noisy is the pump?* All electric pumps will make noise but some are louder than others, which may be important to you if you're wanting to discreetly pump at work.

• *Is the vacuum ('suck') on the pump adjustable?* If it is you can alter how hard it pulls on your nipple to find your own balance between discomfort (if it sucks too much) and very slow collection of milk (if it doesn't suck enough)

• *If it's electric, is it mains or battery or both?* If you are planning on expressing discreetly when out it might be useful for it to be able to run on batteries.

• *How easy is it to clean?* Does it have lots of fiddly bits or is it easy to just dunk in a pot of sterilising solution?

• *How big is it?* This is more relevant if you are planning on taking it out with you.

Finally, it's worth bearing in mind that if you

don't want to buy a breast-pump but think one would be useful you may be able to hire one from your local NCT group or hospital.

Nipple cream
Rating: advisable if breast feeding
Price: £1 to £10 per tube

If you are breast feeding your nipples are an essential piece of equipment that you need to keep in tip-top shape – which can be a challenge given their user is a newborn! Nipple cream is extremely useful in preventing nipples becoming sore and cracked, so a tube is a great investment for any breast-feeding mum. It is also invaluable in rescuing nipples after they've become cracked, if you're not proactive enough to use it prophylactically (like I wasn't.)

It can initially seem quite expensive – the most popular brand sells for around £10 for a small tube – but it does last a long time and usually one tube is enough to see you through breastfeeding one baby.

Bibs

Rating: optional
Price new: £0.50 to £5 each

When a friend gave me a pack of bibs before Sam was born I initially thought they wouldn't be a very useful gift – I was planning on exclusively breast-feeding, and to me bibs were for bottle-fed babies. However, after around 3 months (I'm something of a slow learner) I realised that if Sam wore a bib that would catch his possets/mini-vomits/drool, so instead of having to wash a whole outfit I could just wash a bib! This (retrospectively obvious) idea revolutionised the size of my washing pile!

As with all baby-items there are a range of bib options, and as per other items which is best for you will depend on your, and your baby's, personal preference. Some bibs have plastic backs, some are all cotton, some are a superabsorbent material. Some fasten with poppers, some with Velcro, and some are retro and require tying a bow (which is probably the worst option as they are fiddly and potentially dangerous in terms of baby managing to strangle themselves). One area to pay particular attention to is the neckline - some bibs have a high, padded neck which is excellent for absorbing drips and protecting the top of clothing. Overall, the best option is probably to not buy too many of any one type so you can see which is the best version for you.

Alternatively, you may not want to bother with any at all. At the end of the day a muslin (see Chapter 10 'Keeping Baby and Mum Happy') will work just as well.

Feeding pillow
Rating: optional
Price new: £20 to £50

If you are planning on breast-feeding, a feeding pillow might be helpful to make positioning baby easier and breast-feeding simpler and more comfortable. Some mums swear by them, whilst others get by quite happily by either just using a normal cushion or nothing at all.

If you do decide to buy one, an added bonus is that feeding pillows are excellent for placing around baby when they are learning to sit up to provide a soft landing when they fall!

As with all baby-related purchases I'd recommend checking that the cushion cover is both removable and machine-washable.

Bottle warmer

Rating: optional
Price new: £13 to £50

A bottle warmer was one of the commonest listed 'worst buys' on internet forums – nearly 7 mums listed it as a worst buy for each one that thought it was a 'best buy'. The majority seemed to find that bottle warmers simply took too long to warm a bottle, and the overall conclusion tended to be that a jug of hot water worked as well and was quicker. and to be honest, I've really just included 'bottle warmer' here to prompt you to think about whether you actually need to buy one.

7 Cleaning Baby

Baby bath

Bath Support

Bath thermometer

Baby towels x 2

Baby nail scissors

Olive oil

Baby hair brush

Baby bath
Rating: optional
Price new: £5 to £20

A special baby bath is one of those items that divides parents – some state they couldn't live without one, while others feel buying one was a waste of money as they barely used theirs. On the internet forums it was in fact the most commonly listed 'worst buy', with 77 posts including it on their 'worst buy' lists. However, 29 posts put it on their 'best buy' lists, once again showing how everyone is different!

Of course, a baby bath is not essential – alternative ways to wash baby include using a washing up bowl, the kitchen sink, a clean bucket or your just your usual bath - so if you're short on space or money you might choose not to get one.

The main benefits of buying a baby bath are:
• it can feel 'safer' to use than a bigger bath while you are gaining confidence in bathing your baby
• the smaller size may be less intimidating to baby, meaning they enjoy bath time more
• it needs less water than an adult bath
• if your bathroom is cold you can use the baby bath to bathe baby in a warmer part of your home

If you do decide to buy one there are multiple

variations on the standard baby bath that you might wish to consider, including:

• ***baby baths with a built-in plug,*** which can be helpful if you're weak like me and are planning on using it in your bath as it means you can let the water out rather than having to have the strength to turn the bath over to empty the water

• '***over the top of bath' models*** that sit across the sides of the adult bath, allowing you to bathe baby at a more comfortable level

• '***fold up' baby baths*** to save space/allow easier transport if travelling

• ***inflatable baby baths*** – with the same benefits as fold-up versions

• '***dividers'*** which (as the name suggests) divide the adult bath, turning it into a smaller bath for bath with the benefits of using less water and possibly making baby feel more secure

• '***tummy tubs'*** which look a little like a bucket and are designed to encourage baby to bathe in the foetal position they were in in the womb, which in theory makes bath time more relaxing for them.

Realistically you are unlikely to be using a baby bath beyond around the three month mark as by then baby will be too big for it, so it really is a short-term item that you may choose to forgo. But, if you do decide to buy one you can always take heart in its numerous potential uses 'post baby', such as for teddy bear storage, as a garden planter or even as an 'ice bath' to store cans in during parties in the summer!

Bath support
Rating: optional
Price new: £8 to £20

Bath supports are moulded foam or plastic seats that sit in the bath to 'support' baby (the clue was in the name really) and so leaving your hands more free to wash baby/play with ducks and bath toys. On the internet forums more mums thought these were useful than those that thought baby baths were useful, and in contrast to baby baths, bath supports featured on 'best buy' lists more frequently than 'worst buy' lists!

Benefits of bath supports over baby baths are that they can be used for longer and take up less space, so they may be worth considering if you're feeling anxious about bathing baby but don't fancy buying a baby bath. The main disadvantage is that bath supports limit a baby's ability to splash and wiggle... but if you have a carpeted bathroom and you don't want the floor to get wet this may be an advantage for you!

Bath thermometer
Rating: advisable
Price new: £6 to £16

Babies should be bathed in water that is roughly 37C – too cold and they will be unhappy and start to shiver, too hot and baby will be scolded. The traditional method for checking temperature is to put your elbow into the water. However, if you are like me and completely inept at judging temperature, a bath thermometer is a must-have. Even my husband (who is an infinitely better judge of temperature than me) found having it reassuring, and when you are sleep-deprived it just makes life that little bit easier and safer by removing any guess-work over the temperature.

Bath thermometers vary from basic models that don't tell you the actual temperature and instead just show red or green depending on whether the water is too hot or not, to beautiful versions that can double as room-thermometers and are designed to also be used as bath toys, so if you're going to buy one shop around to find a version that appeals to you.

Baby towels
Rating: optional
Price new: £4 to £19

Babies are very bad at regulating their body temperatures and so start shivering rapidly after coming out of the bath. Since most heat is lost through the head the built-in hoods on baby towels help to instantly minimize heat loss and so decrease the amount of shivering (and hopefully crying!) However, some mums complain these towels are too small to wrap even a newborn baby up snuggly and that baby grows out of them so quickly anyway that they're not worth it, so again its up to you if you think they'd be helpful.

One thing possibly worth bearing in mind is that if you're going to take little one swimming owning at least one towel with a built-in hood would be useful as you can take it with you to the poolside to help warm baby up as soon as they come out of the water.

Baby nail scissors
Rating: advisable
Price new: from £2

Baby's nails grow with surprising speed and quickly become dangerous weapons that they use indiscriminately against your nipples/arms/their own faces. Trimming them is therefore important (if scary) and baby nail scissors make this process a littler easier and less fraught with danger.

Olive oil
Rating: advisable
Price: from around £1

Babies often have patches of dry skin and olive oil is a cheap, safe way to help keep baby moisturized. It is also very good for treating cradle cap, which is another ailment that is unfortunately rather common. And if you find you don't need it you can always use it in your cooking!

Baby hair brush
Rating: advisable
Price: from around £1

A hairbrush with soft bristles is very useful in keeping your baby looking tidy. It can also be invaluable in brushing out flakes from cradle cap after you've used moisturizer or olive oil to loosen them.

8 On the move

Car seat
? base for car seat
**? adapters for car seat to fit
   on pram**
Car mirror
Pram
Baby carrier/sling
Travel cot

Car seat

Rating: essential
Price: : from £33 to £269

A car seat is an absolute essential – many maternity units won't let you leave hospital with your baby without one. It is also an item that should really be purchased new, as a second-hand one may have damage (which will not necessarily be visible) that might weaken it and mean it does not protect your baby in the event of an accident.

When choosing your first car seat you need to buy one that is either Group 0 or Group 0+, which together are known as "Stage 1" seats (note however that "Group 1" seats are not suitable from birth, so make sure you don't get your stage 1 and group 1 seats confused!) The difference between Group 0 and Group 0+ seats is that Group 0 is suitable from birth to around 10kg in weight, while group 0+, while also suitable from birth, can be used up to the slightly heavier weight of around 13kg. If you're like me those weights won't mean much to you at the moment, so to put it into context if you have an 'average' baby boy he will weigh 10kg at around 13 months of age and 13kg by around 28 months of age.

As with all important safety equipment there are specific standards car seats must meet, but if you are buying new from a reputable company it is a given that these standards will be met so that's one less thing to worry about.

So other than making sure the seat is new and suitable from birth, what other things do you need to consider? The main thing I'd advise you to be aware of is how heavy the seats are – being a bit of a weakling I was struggling to lift some of the seats in the shop and that was before there was the added weight of having my baby in it! For this reason alone I'd recommend going to a big store so you can get a 'feel' for the various different carseats, even if you plan to buy one online afterwards.

The other thing you can check when looking at seats in store is how they fasten (although this tends to be very similar for all of them) and how much padding they have, so you can have an idea of both how easy it will be for you to put baby in and how comfortable it will be for baby.

And, obvious though this sounds, make sure the seat you choose fits in your particular car, and in any other cars (grandparents, carers) that you baby may need to be taken in.

Now, although all seats can be secured using the seat belts in the car, you might wish to consider buying a base unit, such as the isofix, which makes putting the seat in and out of the car quicker and easier. A base unit remains in the car all the time and allows the baby seat to be secured simply by 'clicking' into place on top of it, meaning you don't have to fiddle around securing it with seatbelts whenever you go out – a great time and sanity saver, especially if you have a baby like mine who screams hysterically from the moment he is put in his seat until the point the car is in motion (at which point he briefly coos happily before falling asleep!)

The final car seat 'optional extra' you may wish to buy is a set of adapters that allow the car seat to fit onto your pram base. One advantage of this is if you are just making a short trip followed by a little bit of walking around, for example to the supermarket, you can use your car seat as a pram to save having to take the pram too - but remember a baby should never be in a car seat for too long as it is bad for their developing spine. Another advantage of having adapters is that if you live in an area where you park on the road and you may end up parking your car quite a trek from your home it allows you to push baby home in the car seat rather than having to struggle to carry the heavy and unwieldy carseat/baby combo.

Car mirror
Rating: optional
Price: from around £4

Babies have to travel in rear-facing car seats in

the back whilst young. While this may be the safest way, it does make it impossible to see baby when you are driving. A mirror can therefore be useful to provide reassurance/keep an eye on your little one.

The two main types are either one that attaches to the rear window, or one that attaches to the other rear passenger headrest. If you have a hatchback the type that attach to the window tend to fall off with annoying frequency, so if you aren't going to have a passenger in the other rear seat the attach to the rear passenger headrest option may be best.

A limitation of some of these mirrors is that they are small and not of a very high quality, meaning that on using them all you can really see is that your baby is in his carseat. Which you already knew anyway, making it not that useful.

So if you do get one, don't make the mistake I did in buying a small cheap one that attached to the back window in my hatchback car – it kept falling off and since the reflected image was so small and blurry it didn't help me to tell how my baby was doing, so I think I only used it for one car journey. Now admittedly I'd only spent roughly the same amount as a cup of coffee on it, but quite frankly I would have preferred the cup of coffee...

Pram/travel system
Rating: advisable
Price: very variable...

When I was pregnant I remember my friend Lynne, who had a young baby, telling me that choosing a pram was more difficult than picking a new car. I laughed and thought that she was joking... until I started trying to choose one and discovered she was possibly being deadly serious!

I quickly discovered that many prams are now not just prams – they are in fact part of complex 'travel systems' which include a carrycot (= the traditional 'pram'), a pushchair-type component and possibly also an attachable car seat. And when I went into a specialist baby shop to look at these I wondered if my baby-brain had taken me into a car salesroom instead as I listened to the pram (sorry, 'travel-system') salesperson extolling the 'excellent suspension' on one model, the 'range of frame finishes, gloss and matt' on another, the 'wide choice of fabrics' on a third and the 'small turning circle' on a fourth!

So, the first thing to remember before being sucked into the world of pram-buying (complete with its glossy brochures and car-salesman-like advisors) is that unless you have a very small baby they may not be in the 'carrycot' (=traditional pram part) of the pram for very long at all. This is important as if you were thinking of buying a traditional pram that is just a pram you need to be aware that it may well be a big outlay for something that you won't use for long, so you may wish to consider going for a 'travel system' instead. It is also important as if you were already going to buy a travel system you might now wish to consider prioritizing how much you like the system's pushchair-part over it's carrycot-part as it's the pushchair-part you'll be getting the most use out of. Alternatively, if the pushchair-part lies almost flat you might decide not to bother buying the carrycot part of the travel system at all and instead carry baby in a sling/carrier until they are big enough for the pushchair part.

The final reason it's important to pause to think before being beguiled by glossy adverts is that you may decide to not bother buying a pram/travel-system at all and decide instead use a baby sling/carrier until baby is big enough to go into a fold-up pushchair. This option may seem crazy but if you're a fit, active mum and live somewhere hilly/with lots of steps you might find that carrying baby is actually easier than using a pram and just suits your lifestyle better.

If you do decide to get a pram/travel system, I'd suggest considering the following points to help choose the one best for you:

• ***What do you need the pram for?*** This

will help you prioritise what features are important to you – for example, if you are going to be doing lots of off-road walking the suspension will be important, while if it will be used for your weekly shop a big basket underneath will be more of a priority.

• *How big is it?* Will it fit through your front door when up and in your car boot when folded? Some modern prams are surprisingly large - my friend Justine loving refers to hers as 'the tank'. It does have the best suspension of any pram I've seen but I'm not sure it would fit in my car even if I put the back seat down!

• *How easy is it to steer?* How big is it's 'turning circle? Every pram is different and you don't want to end up with one that feels to you like pushing a misbehaving shopping trolley!

• *Does it have suspension?* This is less important if you'll be using it on smooth pavements in town but may be critical if you're going to be on country paths a lot.

• *How easy is it to fold up?* Remember you may be trying to do this while holding a baby in one arm.

• *How heavy is it to carry?* It's no good if you're going to need to take it in your car but it's too heavy for you to lift into the boot alone.

• *Can the pushchair part face both outwards and towards you?* This is useful as when baby is little they'll want the reassurance of seeing you, but once they're bigger you'll be 'boring' and they'll prefer to see where you're going.

• *Does it have a shopping basket?* And how big is it?

• *Can the handle height be adjusted*? This may be important if you and your other half are very different heights.

• *Does it come with a raincover?* Because if it doesn't and you live in the UK you're going to have to pay extra to buy one!

As this is a big purchase, and there are so many variables, make sure you go to a store and try some out to help you decide which one you want, even if once you've decided you start looking for that model on ebay.

Baby carrier/sling
Rating: advisable
Price: £20 to £139

There are three main reasons why a baby carrier/sling is a good investment:

1. *It frees up your hands.* Babies love being carried/held. Which is nice (nothing beats a good baby-snuggle) but can be prohibitive to you getting anything else done, including things that pre-baby

you would have taken for granted, such as making and eating a sandwich or popping some washing in the machine. Using a baby carrier means you can meet your baby's desire to be held whilst also getting things done (which may well also help save your sanity).

2. *It can save your back.* If you have a baby who wants to be carried around all the time eventually your back will start to resent them for it and express this by hurting you. A baby carrier can spread the weight more evenly and so stop your back hurting so much.

3. *It can give you more freedom when out and about.* Taking baby out in a pram means you can't squeeze through gaps or take stairs and will just generally make slower progress than you previously did. However, if you have baby in a carrier/sling you can walk around much like you did before, except with a small person attached to you.

So if you're now sold on the idea of a carrier/sling (and I must confess that while I wasn't pre-baby, post baby I am their biggest advocate) how do you choose one? As with many baby-related things they come in many different forms, ranging from structured 'clip up' ones to wrap-around tie one, with some where baby faces in and others where baby faces out. Deciding which one will be best for you is a personal choice, so the best thing to do is to go to a store which stocks a few different brands so you can try a few and see which feels best.

A few things to bear in mind when choosing include:

• *How will the baby's weight be distributed?* Some carriers/slings have straps on the shoulders and waist to share the load, while others may be just over the shoulders or even just over one shoulder, which may become uncomfortable very quickly as baby gets heavier.

• *What age range is it suitable for?* Some carriers aren't suitable from birth, while others have 'weight limits' meaning they won't be appropriate for use beyond a few months of age.

• *Where is baby carried?* A small baby will need to be carried on the front, but as they grow into a toddler can the carrier be used on a hip/the back as well? And can it face outwards?

• *What position is baby carried in?* There is lots of variation in this, ranging from curled up to upright with all the weight going through their crotch to sitting with legs spread around you.

• *How easy is it to get on and off?* Some carriers involve just a few clicks, others might be more 'wrap like' and require more skill whilst a few are straightforward enough but need considerable flexibility to do up on your own (which is realistically what you'll be doing most of the time.)

• **Can it be washed?** If so is it machine washable? As with all things to do with baby it is likely to get vomit/other bodily fluids on it at some point.

• **Does it have any pockets** built into it/any clips to attach a small bag to?

Travel cot
Rating: optional
Price: £25 to £200

It may seem rather pre-emptive to put a travel cot on the list of things to buy before baby is even born, but the reality is if you are planning on travelling with baby (even if its just to stay with your parents overnight) you are going to need one, and the sooner you buy one the more use you can get out of it. Another good reason for buying one sooner rather than later is that if you purchase one with a built-in bassinet you could potentially use it as a 'day cot' in your living room if you don't have a moses basket you can move around.

If you decide to buy a travel cot, some things to consider are:

• **Does it have a bassinet feature?**
• **How heavy is it?**

• Does it have wheels to help you move it?
• How big is it – both when folded and when up?
• How good is the mattress part?
• Does it have any 'extras' that you'd like, such as built-in changing table, storage pockets or music centre?

You may also wish to consider whether the one you opt to buy could double as a play-pen for when baby gets a bit older - mine became the safe-haven I'd put Sam in with some toys so I could pop to the loo once he began to crawl!

9 Keeping baby (and mum!) happy

Baby bouncy chair

Play mat

Baby swing

Muslins x 10

Toys

Digital thermometer

Baby bouncy chair
Rating: advisable
Price new: £10 to over £100

When I was pregnant I remember thinking I'd never want to put my precious baby down. I imagined that I'd cuddle him whenever he was awake, inhaling his intoxicating new baby smell, and I assumed I'd have plenty of time to get housework and other dull tasks done while he was sleeping in his crib. However, once he arrived I quickly realised my 'cuddle whenever not asleep' plan was doomed: my gorgeous baby (who did indeed possess that fabulous and intoxicating new baby smell) seemed to think that sleep was overrated and that if his tiredness became so extreme he had to submit to sleep there was no way he was going to do so anywhere except on mummy. And boy, if I had the audacity to put him in his crib (whether awake or apparently asleep) he proved to me just how well his lungs could work. I quickly realised that not only was my 'do housework when baby is asleep' plan flawed, but that even achieving basic daily tasks (you know, like going to the loo) was challenging. I needed somewhere where he'd be safe and happy which was not in my arms, and it transpired that for Sam this 'somewhere' was his bouncy chair. Seriously, the bouncy chair was a life-saver (or at least a sanity-saver) – in time it became the only thing Sam would sleep in during the day (apart from on me) and perhaps even more importantly it made it possible for me to have a shower/empty my bladder (thankfully I never reached the point of being quite desperate enough to have to do those 2 at the same time) as I could put Sam in it in the bathroom, where he would do wonders for my self-esteem by giggling at me when I was naked. I could also put him in it in the corner of the kitchen while I made and wolfed down a sandwich, or on the side of the room while I hung up laundry. In short, it enabled me to keep functioning.

I hadn't bothered to buy one before Sam was born (it just hadn't crossed my mind) which retrospectively I find incredible, as it was definitely the best investment we made. But don't just take my word for it - reading the mummy 'best and worst' buy forums it was the item that was listed the most times by mums as their best buy (even beating sleeping bags) with nearly 1 in 5 mums loving theirs enough to put it on their best buy list. It's also worth noting that bouncy chairs can also be helpful for babies who suffer from reflux as they sit them at an angle that helps relieve the pain.

So if you are now persuaded to go and buy one, is there anything you should be aware of? Well, as with most items of baby equipment, bouncy chairs come in a huge range, from basic metal frame covered in material which you can bounce by pressing up and down on it (or by baby wiggling in once he's bigger) to 'all-singing-all-dancing' versions which vibrate, play music, have adjustable backs to allow you to alter baby's angle and have multiple dangling toys attached. Personally, as a mum with a fussy baby, the 'basic' bouncy chair just didn't cut it with him – he wanted the 'massage chair' experience with the vibrate option – but other mums I know have babies who are perfectly happy with the more basic versions. Once again, I'm afraid this is something that you just need to decide which one you think will work best for you.

Play mat/gym
Rating: optional
Price new: £20 to £60

Playmats/play gyms come in an even more dazzling array of varieties than bouncy chairs. Some are literally just colourful mats, while most have padded 'bars' arching over them dangling a range of toys for baby to play with. The mat itself may be very padded, slightly padded, unpadded, have built in squeakers or crackly material or furry bits, and additionally there may be the option of flashing lights or music. In short, the possible variations are just too great to cover, and which one you opt for (if you decide to get one) is likely to basically be down to which you like the look of most!

The reasons for buying one include:

• it gives you another safe place to put down baby

• it can help keep baby amused (and therefore calm and not crying)

• it can encourage baby to reach for things with the dangling toys

• it can be used for 'tummy time', which is when you place baby on their tummy under supervision to encourage muscle development – although the majority of babies I know regard this as a form of torture rather than useful to practice the first step towards crawling...

Around 10% of mummies on the internet forums I read listed playmat/gym as one of their best buys, while 2% disliked theirs enough to put it as a worst buy, so its up to you (as always!) whether you want to buy one. One thing to bear in mind is that although new they can be quite expensive there always seem to be a lot of good-quality ones available second-hand.

The other thing to remember about playmats is depending on the version you buy their constituent parts may be useful even after baby has outgrown it – once Sam was bored of his I cannibalised it and used the mat part to make a fun base for his 'play pen' (which is actually his travel cot, see chapter 8) and attached some of the dangly toys that came with it to his pushchair, so when buying one you could look with one eye to the future to consider what potential it might have beyond a playmat.

Baby swing
Rating: optional
Price new: £25 to £150

Many babies love the gentle motion of being rocked in mummy's arms, but this can become quite tiring (although good for toning down those dreaded 'bingo wing' flabby arms!). If you have a baby who falls in love with being rocked a baby swing can be invaluable, as it allows the gentle rocking motion to continue whilst you can get on with doing other things.

10% of mummies listed the swing as one of their best buys, while around 3% listed it as among their worst. Given that (relatively) not many people buy baby swings this suggests that it is quite a polarizing buy – those that buy one either love it or hate it.

Baby swings tend to be more expensive than other 'entertainment options' (such as bouncy chair or playmat) so it might be a buy to delay until your baby is born and you have a better idea of whether they are likely to like being rocked/swung or not. If you are planning on getting one, the following points are worth considering:

- **Can it swing at variable speeds** to suit your baby's mood?
- **Does it play music?** If so can you alter the volume and do you have a choice of different songs... and are they songs that you can cope with for prolonged periods of time?
- **Does it recline?** Because if you're hoping baby might sleep in it you need one that does.
- **Is the seat cover detachable and machine washable?**
- **Does it just run on batteries or can you plug it in?**
- **What are the minimum and maximum weights baby can be to use it?**
- **How much space does it take up when in use, and how small can it fold down?**

Muslins
Rating: essential
Price new: from 50p each

A muslin square is a type of light cloth which is sometimes described as "a mother's secret weapon" and, if you're anything like me, it will probably become your new best friend once you have a baby as they are so versatile and relatively cheap. It may seem a strange item to put in this section on keeping baby and mum happy, but trust me it is sooooo useful at keeping mummy sane it definitely deserves its inclusion here.

The main use of muslins tends to be in mopping up vomit or protecting clothes/furniture from vomit.

However, other potential uses for the humble muslin cloth include:

- as a comforter for baby (better than a toy as easier to wash and to replace if lost!)
- as a bib
- over the changing mat so it's less cold (and as an added bonus will absorb small wees!)
- to dry baby's bottom after using wipes
- as a temporary sunshade when out with the pram (but note they don't provide UV protection, just shade from the glare)
- tucked into your top while breastfeeding to catch dribbles of milk
- as a temporary changing mat when "out and about"
- as a light cover instead of a blanket over a baby in the summer
- as a "privacy shield" when breastfeeding in public
- as a 'toy' to play peekaboo with
- as a mat for baby to play on

They wash well and dry quickly, but even so you'll likely find you can never have enough, especially if you have a sicky baby. I thought my initial purchase of 16 was plenty but had invested in a further 8 before Sam was a month old!

Another benefit is that any muslins which survive the baby years can be usefully employed as dusters or handkerchiefs afterwards.

In case you're still not convinced, muslins were the third most mentioned items on mums' 'best buy' lists.

Toys
Rating: optional

When your baby is born, they won't really care for anything beyond milk, burps, clean nappies and cuddles, but very quickly toys to entertain/distract become important. Do you really need to buy any toys at all before baby is born? Not necessarily. And advising which to buy is difficult as there are just so many options and different babies like different things – and even the same baby, at different ages, can change dramatically – for example, a singing glowworm toy (squidgy body, light up face) scared Sam and invariably made him cry when he was 2 months old, but by 4 months the same toy was the ultimate solution to his worst crying fits and never failed to soothe him!

Even the trusted internet 'best and worst' buy lists aren't that helpful in me trying to provide some sort of evidence/justification for this section as toys are rarely mentioned, so the list of suggested good buys below is entirely anecdotal based on what has been most used in our home, and in those of my friends.

My suggested toys are therefore:

• *'Traditional' baby rattle with a handle* - good for noise and then good for teething!

• *Big (around 10cm) soft cubes* with pictures on them – great for tummy time play and you don't have to worry about baby falling on them and hurting themselves, as if anything they help break sudden plunges!

• *Sophie La Giraffe* – a rubbery teething toy in the shape of (no surprises here) a giraffe, with a squeaker in the middle. So good that it will be found in the possession of the vast majority of mothers of teething babies, and squeaking it can provide entertainment for smaller babies before it is required as a teether.

• *Plastic links* – great for playing with and teething on.

• *Stacking rings* – brightly coloured plastic rings that stack onto a pole - fun to peer at baby through, place on wrists and again for baby to chew!

In general you'll be able to decide what to buy by seeing which toys your baby likes at baby groups/when visiting friends, and relatives are likely to give toys as gifts too, so buying before baby is born is not essential.

One last thing to mention: soft toys. People love buying these as gifts, so be prepared to have a whole shelf of them gathering dust without you having to buy any yourself. Although you could follow the lead of one my oldest friends who put all the soft toys she had been given to use on a daily basis by using them as props in a unique version of 'Old MacDonald had a Farm', in which alongside the usual pigs and sheep he had bears, pandas and a dragon!

And finally: if you do decide to buy a special soft toy as a comforter, make sure that it is machine-washable (baby slobber can get surprisingly smelly) and that you have at least 2, in case one gets lost.

Digital thermometer
Rating: advisable
Price new: £25 to £40

So a digital thermometer might not be one of the first things you think of buying when you discover you're expecting, but once baby is here one can be invaluable – when Sam was little he frequently seemed flushed and being able to take his temperature reassured me that in fact it was just a healthy glow rather than anything more worrying. And had the thermometer showed his temperature was up, it would mean I would be able to call the GP with a hard number rather than a vague 'he seems a bit hot...'

Ear thermometers are best and are now affordable, and of course will be useful for the whole family for years to come rather than just being useful for baby short-term.

.

10 For mum

Painkillers
Breast pads x 1 box
Maternity pads x 70
'Feeding Survival box'
Breast-feeding clothes

Painkillers
Rating: advisable
Price: variable

I'm not going to dwell on this too much but the fact is childbirth tends to be a tad uncomfortable and so afterwards you may well want something to take the edge off that. Talk to your friendly local pharmacist before the event if you're not sure what to take.

Breast pads
Rating: essential
Price: around 20p per disposable pair

I was utterly surprised by the somewhat shocking transformation of my breasts from things that were easily contained within a bra to potentially dangerous weapons that sprayed milk from my nipples a little like the fembots in that Austin Power's movie sprayed out bullets. If you are unprepared for this you will end up with spreading damp patches on your tops which visitors will struggle to avert their eyes from (which is embarrassing for both you and them!) Breast pads are therefore fairly essential in the beginning, whether or not you are planning on breast feeding, because although you may know your plan is formula feeding your breasts won't and will still busy themselves with becoming a milk factory.

You can get either disposable or washable breast pads, with the usual pros and cons of cost versus convenience. If you buy disposable ones, look for big sticky tape areas on the backs else they tend to end up scrunched up in your bra, which means you'll have spreading damp patches and a strange silhouette!

How many pads you need will depend partly on whether you are planning on breast feeding or not – initially you'll probably need 2 or 3 pairs a day regardless, but once your breasts have settled down you'll just need a pair a day if you're breastfeeding or none at all if you're not. It's also worth noting that breast pads are a little like nappies in as much as you might find the first brand you try doesn't work for you, so I'd suggest just buying a box to start with.

Maternity pads
Rating: essential
Price: from 10p each

Maternity pads are different from normal sanitary wear in that they are softer and have a smooth surface (so they won't catch on any stitches you may have) and are longer, as the blood may be coming from a, ahem, slightly different distribution than a simple menstrual period.

Bleeding after childbirth can be surprisingly heavy and it's not uncommon to get through 10 pads a day for the first week or so and to then carry on bleeding (but less heavily) for several more weeks. It is therefore a good idea to stock up on at least 70 maternity pads to get you through the initial post-childbirth period when you might not feel up to going out to get more, because lets be honest this is not an item your average male is going to feel comfortable perusing the supermarket aisle for and would definitely not be keen on asking for assistance in finding, meaning if you send them out for some you may find they return instead with a box of chocolates, a sheepish look and the excuse of "ummm they didn't have any"!

Feeding survival box
Rating: advisable

However you plan to feed baby, but particularly if you plan to breast feed, you will quickly discover that the position you are in when you start the feed is the one you are stuck in for quite some time. Since in the early days feeds can be epically long you may well find that while baby is sating himself on your lovely milk you may start to feel a bit pekish yourself. Except you are stuck on the sofa with a latched baby. You may also realize you are ridiculously thirsty, or you need to wipe your nose, or that the TV show that is on is boring you, or your mobile is ringing and you left it in the other room... again, all tough because baby is latched and in the early days disturbing baby during feeding is more hassle than it's worth.

So what you need is a 'feeding survival box' within arms reach. It took me a while to get this (as I've mentioned before, I can be a surprisingly slow learner, especially with the addition of baby brain) but eventually I realised that my days were a lot more pleasant if I kept in a little box (or you could use a tray) next to me with the following:

- Chocolate bar, granola bar, banana or apple
- Can or bottle of drink
- Tissues
- Remote control
- Book (although a kindle would've been easier)
- Mobile phone

I'd definitely recommend seriously considering making up a 'survival box' to your own specification, because anything that makes life easier is worth its weight in gold in those early weeks.

Breast-feeding clothes
Rating: advisable, but NOT the special ones...

If you are planning to breast-feed, you do NOT need to buy any special clothes. Yes, I know all the major baby-stores have rails of clothes marketed 'for breast-feeding mums' but you really don't need them. Basically, they are just normal clothes with slits in strategic positions which allegedly make breast-feeding easier and more subtle as you can poke breast through hole. The problem is that you'll have a bra to sort out under these clothes as well, and the slits are never quite in the right place, and overall you'll probably decide fairly quickly that it's easier to just adopt the 'vest-top under normal-top' approach. The 'vest-top under normal-top' approach just involves you wearing (as the name suggests) a vest top under any 'normal' top so when you need to feed you whip the normal top up and pull the vest top down, allowing you easy access to sort out your bra and then letting you feed baby with minimal skin exposed (good in winter for keeping warm and at any time of year subtleness). This approach doesn't require a new wardrobe as you just use existing tops, but your vest tops do tend to get stretched. If you like the look of the specialist breast-feeding tops, by all means buy some, but as my friend Nic lamented "they were rubbish and now I've just got all these tops with porn holes in them." The other thing to be aware of if you do decide to buy 'special' breast-feeding clothes is to check they are machine washable. I know this may seem utterly incredible but some breast-feeding clothes, particularly the more expensive 'designer' type ones, are hand wash only. So unless you have a live-in maid for laundry be wary of these as baby is likely to get milk/vomit on them frequently.

10 Things to avoid buying

It's quite hard to write a section on what to avoid buying as if you read any internet mummy forum, or discuss with any of your friends who are mummies, you'll find many baby items are like marmite: people either love them or hate them. However, the following items seem to consistently feature as regrets, so here is a top 10 of things to think carefully before investing in:

1. Top and tail bowl – this is a bowl divided into 2 halves, the idea being you use one half for washing baby's face and the other for washing baby's bottom. My top and tail bowl got used for one week before my pregnancy brain receded slightly and I realised I could use a normal bowl (which was smaller and more convenient to fill) and just wash Sam's face first and then his bottom. Around 6% of mums on the internet forums were equally disillusioned with their top and tail bowls and put it on their worst buy list.

2. Cot bumpers – yes, they may look pretty but what many mums-to-be don't realise when buying them is that they increase the risk of cot death... which they become aware of after the helpful midwife tells them after baby is born, which means they never use the bumpers and they just take up space in a cupboard gathering dust.

3. Bottle warmer – electrical bottle warmers are purchased by many mums but, judging from the overwhelmingly negative comments on the best and worst buy threads, are then often rarely used, with a jug of boiling water being repeatedly mentioned as an easier alternative. 9% of mums felt annoyed enough about having one to put it on their 'worst buy' list and for every nine mums who put it on the worst buy list just one said it was a best buy.

4. Scratch mits – scratch mits are a great idea in theory, as newborns do seem overly keen on making their skin look like they've offended the vicious neighbourhood cat, but scratch mits are only any good if they stay on. And in general they don't, and while not designed for the purpose baby socks often work better.

5. Baby booties/shoes – I concede baby shoes look exceedingly cute and I was delighted to be given several pairs, including some particularly adorable koala ones, but without exception they either fell off spontaneously or were 'helped' off by Sam. I think the koala ones were relegated from 'item of footwear' to 'bedroom ornament' after I'd put them back on around 20 times in one trip to the postbox. Which, considering I can see aforementioned postbox from my living room window, was an awful lot of times. Internet 'worst buy' lists tended to give similar tales of shoe-related woe, so it may be best to spend your money on a less frustrating purchase. One alternative to consider might be socks that look like shoes – Sam had several pairs in different colours which really finished his outfits off beautifully when he got a bit bigger, and were far easier to keep on than shoes. If you have a baby girl you could also consider the tights you can find that are designed to look like they have shoes on the bottom too.

6. Toiletries – babies' skin is delicate and prone to eczema. Many mummies therefore end up either using no toiletries at all in bathwater, or needing various moisturisers as recommended by their GP. Net result is often bottles of unopened baby shampoo alongside barely used baby bubble bath.

7. Soft toys – as mentioned in chapter 9 ('Keeping Baby and Mum Happy') lots of soft toys are given as gifts and then end up just sitting collecting dust on a shelf without you needing to buy any yourself. If you do decide to buy one that you hope will become your baby's comforter, check if it's machine-washable and then consider buying a spare in case it gets lost!

8. Nappy bin – this is definitely a 'marmite' item: nappy bins were the third most commonly listed 'worst buy', but were also so beloved by other mums that for every 10 who listed it as a worst buy,

6 mums listed listed it as a best! See Chapter 5 ('Changing Baby') for a more complete discussion.

9. Baby bath – this was the item that would have won the internet forum 'wooden spoon' award as it was the item most frequently mentioned on the 'worst buy' lists. If you haven't already read Chapter 7 ('Cleaning Baby') have a peek now for further details plus ideas of what you could do with a baby bath other than use it as a baby bath.

10. Moses basket – this was the item which came runner-up to baby bath on the 'worst buy' lists, but it was also another marmite-eqsue item as for every 2 mums who thought it was a 'worst' buy, 1 thought it was a 'best' buy. Chapter 4 has a more complete discussion of the pros and cons

11 Where to buy things

Although buying things ready for baby may at first glance look ruinously expensive, it doesn't need to be (and hopefully the number-crunching in Chapter 2 also helped reassure you!)

Firstly, remember that you may well not need to actually buy things – friends/relatives who have completed their families will likely be more than happy to de-clutter their homes by giving you items such as baby baths or sacks of clothes, and even people you don't know that well may offer you things they no longer need when they find out you're expecting – for example, I am indebted to one of my colleagues who I barely knew but who gave me a cot, carrier and a big bag of clothes (thank you Sarah G!)

Friends and family are also likely to want to buy presents for your new arrival, so there's nothing wrong with hinting that a certain thing would be very much appreciated (and this may also help avoid you ending up with shelves full of stuffed toys...)

Another possible way to get things for free is to use freecycle (www.freecycle.org), which is a website where people advertise things they no long want and are willing to give away for free if you can collect them.

Inevitably however you will have to buy some things, but remember that the majority of items do not need to be bought new. Babies grow out of things so fast that many second hand items are pristine, and in some cases may be second-hand but unworn/never used – for example, I have clothes I bought for Sam that I put in a drawer ready for when he got bigger and then completely forgot about them, and when by chance I found them again he had got too big!

The only exceptions to second-hand being acceptable are car-seats, which should always be new due to the potentially fatal implications of a sub-standard second hand one, and mattresses for cots/cribs, which should ideally be new as old mattresses are associated with an increased risk of cot death.

Sources of second-hand baby things to buy include:

• Internet sites such as e-bay.co.uk or gumtree.com
• Charity shops
• Car boot sales
• Adverts in local papers
• Adverts in newsagents/supermarket windows
• 'Nearly new' baby sales, organized by groups such as the NCT

Even if you buy things new, with careful shopping you can still avoid maxing out your credit card. Big supermarkets often sell baby clothes and other essentials that are of reasonable quality and wash well at very competitive prices. The big specialist baby shops (such as Mamas and Papas and Mothercare) tend to be more expensive, but if you are able to bide you time you may be able to find online discount codes to make them more affordable. Small local baby shops can often also have unexpected bargains. And as I pointed out in Chapter 2, if you buy all the 'essential' and 'advisable' items new but as cheaply as possibly the total cost is likely to be around £615, falling to £280 if you just bought 'essential' items

So... happy shopping, and good luck!

Epilogue

I started writing this while breastfeeding Sam, using one hand to type whilst the other cradled his tiny head. Now I can only work on the finishing touches when he's asleep in his cot, as there is no way I'd be able to type with my gorgeous little explorer awake and trying to 'help' me! He has already outgrown many of the items in this book and they are carefully bagged in the loft in case of further siblings, and it feels like a lifetime ago that I was wandering round shops feeling utterly overwhelmed and totally confused as to what I needed, when in fact it was only a year ago. So all those people who tell you 'they grow up so fast'... well, it appears they're right!

I hope this book has been helpful to you and you now feel ready to 'buy for baby' with confidence. Best of luck with everything and, although it's a cliché, it really won't be long until you too are packing up items that your baby has outgrown!

Finally, I'd love to hear your feedback about this book - please do email me (sarahhudsonuk@gmail.com) with suggestions for changes/additions, or just to say hello!

Sarah Hudson

19779426R00074

Printed in Great Britain
by Amazon